Free Your Body of TUMORS and CYSTS

by Rev. Hanna Kroeger, Ms.D

4th Printing February 2010

Copyright 1997
by
Hanna Kroeger Publications

ISBN 978-1-883713-18-8

TABLE OF CONTENTS

INTRODUCTION
Cancer

The word "cancer" has such a terrible sound. It is a death sentence in six letters. It is an end of all your dreams. It ruins your family. It ruins springtime and the fall. You can't see the beauty of the flowers any longer, nor the sky with the sailing clouds. The helping hand you push away, because you gave in to six small letters, "cancer." The "C" is twice in this word, just to make it sharp and pointed, irritating and hurting. With its hooks, it penetrates your mind, and like a fish hook in your flesh, this hook cannot be pulled out of your mind easily. It sticks in your mind—"cancer, I have cancer."

Cancer has become one of the most common diseases in America. Every third person has it, and statistics go as far as to say every second person has it. We should be used to hearing the word "cancer" without fear. But, instead, the fear phantom increases with every case diagnosed. This fear syndrome is paralyzing to our inborn defense mechanism. We just give in. Like a mouse is paralyzed for fear when a snake comes close, so, most of us are paralyzed when the verdict is given that *you* have cancer.

We go to our desks and start cleaning out. We put our estates and affairs in order. In our minds, we say good-bye to all plans and dreams we have for the future. And we retreat into a shell that screams, "Don't touch me, I am doomed."

If this happens to *you*, turn around and uplift your life. Go to the dress shop and spend some money on a pink or rose-colored dress, and then get fitted for some high-heeled shoes. Know that you can overcome your resentments and your fear syndrome.

Take a mild, herbal sleeping pill until you are over the first shock. Then start creating your life all over again, new and beautiful.

In every case, when your health has deteriorated to the point of diagnosis, you belong under the guidance of a physician. Besides that, you cannot go on undermining your health with all the wrongdoings you have been doing over the years. Rebuilding your health is your problem, not your physician's. The physician helps you to eliminate illness, but you, and you alone, can rebuild your health.

Health is the most precious possession you, personally, can have. You cannot buy it, you have to work at it. You have to sacrifice for it. Health is your heritage, your freedom from illness. Just as the citizens of a nation have to work and sacrifice for the precious gift of freedom, to hold it and keep it, so the individual has to work on the precious heritage of freedom from illness. You work on it by educating yourself, changing your diet and life-style, changing your outlook to see the purpose of life and by believing in the universal law that "as a man soweth, so will he reap."

Editors note: Hanna wrote this book in 1997. Since then, new studies have been made available encouraging the necessary progress of knowledge. Time moves ever forward and this book is intended to show Hanna's thoughts about research and finding solutions to some tough problems, while guiding the reader toward the same goals.

CHAPTER I

TRADITIONAL CONCEPTS
Different Theories on Cancer

Theory I
Cancer is a Disease of Fermentation and Oxygen Deficiency

According to Nobel Laureate, Dr. Otto Warburg, "The prime cause of cancer is the replacement of the respiration of oxygen in normal body cells by a fermentation of sugar." Dr. Warburg adds that cells that aren't able to derive the oxygen and nutrients essential to energy production can only do *one* thing: *SWITCH OVER TO SUGAR FERMENTATION, OR DIE!!* Dr. Warburg won the Nobel prize for his discovery that cancer is a disease of *defective cellular respiration.* He has shown that cancer cells generate an abundance of lactic acid because of this partial anaerobic glycolysis. In short, Dr. Warburg says cancer is caused by the lack of oxygen at the cellular level.

Theory II
Immune Systems Dysfunction

Science has known for years that cancer patients have a weakened immune system and that a healthy immune system has the ability to destroy DNA damaged cells.

Dr's. Stephen Levine and Parris Kidd have identified this defense system and the cell's ability to adapt to oxidative stress through the glutathione cycle. All sorts of chemicals create free radicals, including endocrine hormones that circulate as a result of stress. These free radicals can stretch the capabilities of the antioxidant defense system to the limit and ultimately render it defenseless if vital nutrients aren't replaced. Before this happens those doctors have found that the antioxidant defense system fails in an attempt to adapt to increased utilization of key nutrients. This causes uncontrolled free radical damage with its cross linking, immune dysfunction and chemical hypersensitivity.

Dr. Hans Nieper, M.D., offers this refreshing approach to repair the immune system:

1. activation of the thymus function
2. activating the immune system
3. activating the enzymatic action of the pancreas

Dr. Nieper gives trypsin bromelain chymotrypsin therapy for thymus gland. Also:

> zinc orotate
> calcium orotate
> magnesium orotate

Dr. Nieper says that protein has to be digested and that the protein layer around the cancer cell has to be broken down. He points out when the magnesium level in the blood gets down it shows *immune system fatigue*. Dr. Nieper says that all people with cancer involvement need 200,000 units of vitamin A. The best source is seven ounces of carrot juice, three to four times a day. One tablespoon of whipped cream should be added.

Theory III

Faulty Cell Division

Until he was in his late teens, Albert Szent-Györgyi's family thought he was retarded. But he went on to become one of the world's most honored scientists. Now, at the age of eighty-three and after years of research, he has evolved a theory which may solve the deadly mystery of cancer. Dr. Szent-Györgyi calls his discovery the "electronic theory of cancer." It is based on understanding how cells divide and how this process goes wrong to produce wildly dividing and growing "sick" cells—cancer. Because electrons make cells move, they are the key to understanding cell division. Unlike other cancer researchers who are concentrating on the cause of the disease—there are many causes, from viruses to food additives—Dr. Szent-Györgyi focuses on the cell. "You cannot cure what you do not understand. To fix an automobile engine, first you must know how it works," he says. While enormously complex in detail, in essence, his theory is simple. It is based on how cells grow. Cancer is a distortion of this growth, or wild, uncontrolled division of cells. Division is movement; the agent of movement is the electron. Cells are constantly moving between two states. One is a state of proliferation or division. The other is a resting state. When a cell gets stuck in the first proliferating state, as it will if its electronic moving system is out of order, it will divide uncontrollably and the result will be a cancerous growth. "What makes the cell pathological is that it cannot find its way back to the resting state," Dr. Szent-Györgyi says. If a way can be found to introduce electronic mobility into a cancerous cell to move it out of the wild growth state and into the resting state, it could be the eventual answer to cure or prevention of the disease.

In his address at the Boston University School of Medicine Symposium, Dr. Szent-Györgyi dramatically demonstrated a key element in his theory—that certain proteins can carry electrons. He showed a test tube with a yellow liquid, the color indicating that it was not a "semi-conductor" of electrons. But then he showed a second tube. It was an identical liquid, but the color had been changed, by adding a chemical solution, to a dark, opaque red. Some proteins then are semi-conductors.

"The human body," Dr. Szent-Györgyi says, "is a better machine than we think. It is only when we treat it badly that it fails. Benefits from vitamins are not known for perhaps years after we start taking them," he says, "and then we do not know why we feel good."

Another reason for his hearty old age is that he loves his work—research—and the fight against cancer gives him a strong opponent. It has made him, he says, a "happy man."

Theory IV

Cancer is a Fat-Protein Problem

Dr. Johanna Budwig has a different approach to cancer. She said cancer is a fat-protein problem. Dr. Budwig is the world's leading expert on the therapeutic uses of oils, especially flaxseed oil, also called linseed oil.

She recommends oils and cottage cheese to all her cancer cases with phenomenal results. For years I wondered why such a simple remedy can have such super outstanding results.

I learned that with this formula the body can make its own interferon. What are interferons? Interferons are proteins which are manufactured in the cells when the human body is under attack of fungi or viruses. Interferons "interfere" with the ability of both fungi and viruses to multiply in the body.

There seems to be several interferon proteins. The most outstanding is Interleukin-2-. This particular one is used in kidney tumors and in the management of brain tumors. It also seems to depress the formation of new tumors through metastasis. In fact interferon and Interleukin-2- is a weapon against cancer.

Dr. Budwig registers outstanding results in the management of cancer with the use of her formula of "cottage cheese and oil." This formula provides the body with fuel to make its own interferon and its own Interleukin-2-.

This also is the best prevention against cancer in general. Make one of her recipes twice a week and you will be blessed. Here are some recipes which are tasty and helpful.

> 5 tablespoons of almond oil
> or apricot oil
> or walnut oil
> (Dr. Budwig uses flaxseed oil)

This formula makes interferon in your body. Interferon is needed to combat cancer.

Dr. Budwig said: "Cancer patients have to eat and starve the tumors." She takes raw cottage cheese called "quark" and adds cold pressed oils to it. With this the starved cells are supplied with an oxygen rich product. Even though they never met, her findings coincide with Dr. Szent-Györgyi's research.

Both precious physicians say that certain proteins can carry electrons which are vital for the health of the starving cells. With raw oil Dr. Budwig adds another important factor, "Vitamin F," which also becomes an oxygen carrier to the starving cells.

ATTENTION!

Two years ago I received a letter from a Health Research Foundation that we are approaching a time when 50% of the American population will have "cancer" tumor disease. The time is the year 2000. Physicians work overtime to help. You have to realize that many tumors grow without giving much pain and many of us don't know what happens to their bodies. Some are so big that surgery is the immediate solution, rather than find out why. Following is a letter which made me cry bitterly.

Dear Friend,

I am asking for your urgent help on behalf of all innocent little children who have cancer. Over

4,000 kids are now being seen by St. Jude Children's Research Hospital. And thousands more will develop cancer this year.

Thank you for caring,
Richard C. Shadyac
National Executive Director

P.S. I hope that your own family never suffers the tragedy of losing a child to an incurable disease. At St. Jude Hospital, we're fighting to conquer these killers, and one day someone in your own family may live because we succeed.

As Professor Brauchle could heal leukemia in seven days—So can you.
As Professor Brauchle healed cysts in fourteen days—So can you.
As American Indians heal hard tumors in 3 days—So can you.

With God All Things Are Possible!

CHAPTER II

NEW CONCEPTS
Of Tumor Forming Diseases

Natural medicine offers us a variety of healing alternatives, but just as you must be specific with the types of tools you use in your employment, we must also be specific in the type of natural medicine we will use to treat your cysts or tumors. Thankfully, nature offers us many natural ways to help, each with its own specific mode of action.

Cancer: The New Concept

There are several kinds of tumor-forming diseases. We are used to referring to cysts like cancer, which eliminates the truth to our research.

There are three kinds of fungi which make tumors.

1. The hard, firm tumor (fungus).
2. Maduromycosis, a tumor-forming fungus from India.
3. Prostate cancer caused by a fungus.

There are four kinds of viruses which can form tumors.

1. Papilloma.
   a. Papilloma combined with Epstein-Barr.
2. Epstein-Barr with herpes.
3. Herpes virus with another virus.
4. Retrovirus.

Search for Truth

Here is the story of my life's work. A story so real, so dramatic, and now 38 years later, 38 years of anguish and suffering, I dare to put this story to paper.

"You cannot go to school unless you are inoculated with the polio vaccine." This was told to my children and many others in the school district of Boulder, Colorado.

My children loved school, especially the youngest one, who was in the third grade, and she begged me to take her to the place of inoculation. She was proud that she could return to school, the next day. The third day, after her return to school, she had a severe headache and from then on, the school visits became a torture and a total fiasco.

Looking back, all of us were in total trust and confidence toward the medical establishment, and we searched our hearts if we the parents were to blame.

The disaster came with unbelievable power. With sicknesses we had never seen before. Not everyone was hit, but I soon found out that the intelligent children of our nation were hit the most.

Soon convulsions set in. Whatever we owned went to the doctor's office, the hospital, the medication, and my little girl got worse and worse.

One afternoon, an overworked physician shouted, "If you bring her one more time, we will place her in an institution for the mentally retarded." I felt paralyzed. I sat in the office, my mouth open, all hope was gone. Now I say, "thank you physician, you put me on my own two feet."

God helps those who help themselves.

After this incident, I looked around. I found that other parents became increasingly concerned about their children's behavior. We parents talked it over to compare and to find out what had happened.

It was summertime. Up in the mountains the so-called "flower children" gathered. They came from everywhere, New York, Los Angeles, San Francisco, and they were from all walks of life. There were doctors' and lawyers' youngsters who did not groom their hair nor wash their hands. They would injure the business of their parents.

"Let them have their own experience and then they will come home" was the slogan at that time. The churches closed the doors against them. The society laughed and made fun of them and they were so sick.

The worst were the nights. I experienced these terrible nights with my own child. Chilled, full of fear, screaming from despair, fever and nausea. For hours, I held my daughter in my arms until she relaxed and slept.

I thought of all the other youngsters. Two youngsters sleeping together in one sleeping bag just to keep warm and off-set the fear, the fever, the despair.

The flower children left for warmer climates but in the coming year, it was worse. One time I asked them not to smoke marijuana because of the danger of destroying the brain stem. The answer was "can't we feel good and be ourselves once or twice a week?" The smoke helped them to feel better. After that, I never said a single word about marijuana. Is that why marijuana is used? They were sick, as my child was sick, and they got worse month after month. My child had a home, and my child had us, who cared, kept her warm, and clean. How about the others in the streets, in the mountains living on rice and bananas, bananas and rice?

What Had Happened

In the late-fifties of this century, thousands of little Rhesus apes were shipped to America. They were delivered by the truckloads to laboratories. With long needles their little kidneys were pierced and the deathly polio virus was injected. The little animals became deathly ill. The kidney decomposing with puss and decay. On the heights of their suffering the Rhesus apes were killed and the puss extracted. This was injected into fertile eggs and after a few days the famous Salk Vaccine was ready to be injected into our children's bloodstreams. Many vaccines are made that way; however, here entered the tragedy. The polio virus was dead but no one knew and no one checked that this vaccine slipped in a little virus which is only known to be present in apes.

This ape virus has the scientific name of Simian 40, in short Sim 40. It is a retrovirus, an RNA virus.

Sim 40 is harmless to apes, but when entered into the bloodstream of our children the disaster started.

The big business, the huge propaganda machine, the praise, the advertisement subdued the cries of the parents whose children were suddenly hit with:

fear

lack of cleanliness

anguish

failing physical health

failing mental health

depression

laziness

hatred toward parents and teachers

low grade temperature

listlessness

meningitis

Many more behavioral symptoms which were not present before the vaccine was given. Many physicians realized very soon that something went wrong with the inoculations. To avoid more troubles for their patients they injected sterile water until they knew what was going on, and the propaganda machine became occupied with other things.

Sim 40 had never been in human blood before, and all at once, millions of Americans had it. Sim 40 is a retrovirus which is found in apes, sheep, cattle, and mice. It is an RNA virus. It is a virus that can change according to the environment it is bathed in, and also the amount of life energy or lack of life it gets. Lentivirus is also an RNA virus.

Many of these people are now between 40 and 50 years of age. Many have seen the horror of mental institutions.

Many committed suicide. Many have seen jails from inside and many just exist.

The acute stage of this virus is over; however, it is not dead. The second episode is now showing up. Many, many children, also folks between 40 and 60, senior citizens who never had the first inoculation of polio vaccine, the one which brought on the tragedy, now have Sim 40 in their system. It hides in the spinal fluid, in the nervous system, and they feel tension in the back of their necks and between their shoulder blades. According to medical textbooks, veterinarian textbooks and according to the research done at C.U., Sim 40 is an RNA virus. That means that it goes into the nervous system.

Of all the viruses, retroviruses are the most feared of all because they can stay dormant for many, many years. They will strike whenever the system becomes low in energy.

In spite of all our doings, our daughter got worse and worse. She was 15 now. She had been diagnosed as lymphosarcoma, lympho-leukemia, hepatitis C, swollen belly and blindness. Death was close.

I called Dr. Burwell and asked her what I should do. She answered and it was the right answer. "Let her go, she suffered so much." So, I was sitting at her bedside, holding her little, white hand in mine. I had placed a red rose on her chest so she could leave more easily, and I whispered the childhood verses she knew.

She then stretched and she was gone.

I closed my eyes and said the Lord's prayer. I came to the end and looked at her white sunken face. There it was, a tear, first in her right eye, then in her left. I moistened her dry lips with a cotton sponge and waited. She moved one finger, then one hand. She then opened her mouth and wanted to say something. I waited and prayed. All of a sudden, she asked "Mother what is a mission?" "A mission," I said, "is a promise to God to do something for Him."

Somewhat later she told me, "I was in a beautiful place, lavender, blue, and white. Many people were standing or sitting, and whoever raised their hand was lifted up to Jesus who was in front. It was so peaceful, and I lifted up my hand, but a voice said, 'you have not fulfilled your mission, go back.'"

"Honey, let us fulfill this mission together," I said. "Let us work hard. Our Lord spoke to you that is holy to both of us."

Weeks of despair, weeks of suicidal tendencies. We couldn't leave her alone. She stabbed herself with dull kitchen knives. She went to the lake to drown herself. "I don't want to stay alive, I want to go to the light," was her daily prayer. Looking back, it was a nightmare, a total nightmare. Weeks went by and she gained strength. Her seizures became less frequent. Her eyesight returned, her hearing improved. My daily prayer was "Oh lord, please show me the mission which we have to fulfill." And, He, our Lord, did show us. It was a battle of 30 years to find the truth, to find the answer. Bits and pieces of knowledge filtered through.

The terrible times of flower children and suicidal youngsters were over. Many young people never went back to school. They could not think. They could only do manual labor for 4 to 5 hours and, exhausted, they lay on their cots for hours and hours. When they were overworked, fever and chills set in. No appetite, no strength. The youth and people of our time are the carriers of this terrible virus.

The retrovirus, an animal virus, not recognized, not understood, and not an ounce of medication to help.

The total tragedy hit me, and I still have not forgotten because I realized totally and absolutely, deep in my heart, that this is the mission our Lord talked about.

CHAPTER III

TUMORS

Fungus Tumors

Self-Examination for Fungus Tumors

The following method which is taught in America is a tremendous breakthrough in detecting oncoming cancer 2 years before a tumor is formed.

Take the first morning urine in a celluloid cup. (Not a foam cup). Cover it with one layer of toilet paper and place it in a dark place. In the evening set the celluloid cup in your refrigerator (lowest shelf). Secure it so that no one will disturb it. The next morning pour out the urine. Where air and urine touched, there will be a fatty waxy ring in the cup if fungus cancer is present in your system.

Examine yourself every six months.

Self-Examination Taught in England and Denmark

Sterilize a pin. Prick one finger tip. When the blood comes with a pearl, you are healthy, when it smears, change your diet and lifestyle. When the drop runs and more than several drops come out from one prick in a thin stream, have an examination by a physician, change your diet, get well quickly, and thank God for this knowledge.

Hard Tumors

The hard tumor is a fungus tumor. It appears as hardened lumps in any part of the body. It is the most feared of all lumps, because it is difficult to detect and there is no medicine for it on the market.

An American Indian showed me an unbelievable technique. It is fabulous. It is a dream come true. For food they advised the 4 day American Indian diet. I personally add herbs packed in capsules, as in the following herbal combinations:

1. Blood Toner®
   yellow dock
   cramp bark
   yarrow
   milkweed
   plantain
   tansy
   organic tobacco

2. FNG Care™
   alfalfa seed
   blessed thistle
   goldenseal root

The poison that feeds this kind of growth is the poison the roundworm created. Also watch for blood flukes which are often found in this type of disease.

An American Indian Healing Method for Fungus Tumors

I had the unbelievable fortune to see American Indians heal tumors.

They also heal their tumor patients with stones and I found out that they are magnetic stones. They do the following:

The loadstones—magnetic stones are hit with one stroke "to make them active." The person is laid on a cot on the floor. The stones are placed around the person while the Indians make sure that the part that is hit comes close to the body. They place one stone to the head, one on each side of the body and one on the inside of each foot.

A ceremony starts with sage and feathers, with dancing and asking the Great Spirits to remove all dark forces attached to the body. All night the person has to lay like this. They said they have to lay there 3–4 nights as demonstrated. By looking closer I found that it is the Northpole, the negative side, that came close to the body,and they said that the negative tumor is influenced by it.

We do not have loadstones but we have magnets. Why should we not use them? Place 350-1200 Gauss magnets around the body so that the north side, the negative side, touches the body as the Indians do. It takes only 47 hours of treatments to influence the negative tumor. We could try couldn't we?

We also could try antifungal herbs and herb mixtures as the Indians showed us. What harm could be done? Absolutely no harm. These herbs are safe particularly in the minute amounts they are used.

If you do not want to be tied down for three days, a young man invented the following method:

Negative side of magnet on head.
Negative side of magnet on inside of wrists.
Negative side of magnet on inside of ankles.
Magnets are to remain on body for 47 hours.

NOTE: Do not wear magnets while sleeping and always remove magnets if you are feeling fatigued or lightheaded.

How to Place Magnets

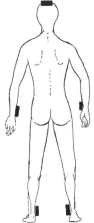

North Side (Negative) on Body for 47 Hours

Quaw Bark

Quaw Bark is the inner bark of an American tree. The American Indians used it for centuries to enhance the healing power of their mixtures. Quaw Bark has the same healing property that has been documented in Brazilian Pau D'Arco. When grown in America, we can utilize its vibration readily.

This bark is used as an anti-fungal and for fighting viral infections as well as having claims to giving strength, stamina, endurance and building the immune system.

Asparagus

"Eating cooked asparagus overcame proven cases of fungus tumors," declared Karl B. Lutz, biochemist, in a letter published in Prevention Magazine. Use fresh, steamed asparagus, or asparagus canned without pesticides or preservatives, from Health Food Stores, Green Giant or Stokeley. Never use raw asparagus. Blend in blender at high speed, he advised. Eat four full tablespoons of asparagus twice daily, morning and evening, hot or cold. The patients usually show improvement in 2 to 4 weeks, he said, and he asked that all who try it send him a report.

Here is one report. A gentleman about 76 years of age developed cauliflower cancer on the ears which appeared thick, crusted and white in color. He was scheduled for surgery but decided to give asparagus a try. In 3 weeks all of it was gone. Pink, healed, amazing.

Concord Grapes/Grape Juice

Concord grapes and Concord grape juice also are known to work against the fungus. If you do not like it, soak dark raisins (currants are best) and drink the juice and eat the soaked raisins.

People with Worms

This kind of tumor carries roundworms. Roundworms are very poisonous and this poison adds to the miserable conditions people are in. See Dr. Hulda Clarke's book on Wormwood Combination.

Herbs in the Management of Fungus Tumors

The Indians are known to have very little cancer. So, I investigated it. It is not the diet because they eat more white sugar and more white bread than any other members of the American continent. But they know herbs and they are the best herbalists.

The Indians gathered the following herbs and made a tea. The formula is also available as an herbal combination.

Blood Toner®
yellow dock
cramp bark
yarrow
milkweed
plantain
tansy
organic tobacco

Milkweed is a North American herb called bloodhoney that is not found in other parts of the world and milkweed is very dear to the Indians. So is tobacco very dear to them and they offer it to their deity. Another tribe took:

FNG Care™
alfalfa seed
blessed thistle
goldenseal root

Both of these 2 herbal combinations taken together show relief to a fungus ridden body. (They are also described above under the *Hard Tumors* section.)

All Indian tribes are aware that tumor victims have parasites and they make sure that these scavengers are removed. They use different kinds of herbs. One Indian lady told me, "Mother cancer in bowels, daughter cancer somewhere else." You have to know that American Indians are born with the 6th sense open clairvoyant, clairaudiant. We have to acquire this through long hours of dedication and meditation.

The Indian observations are so accurate. The Herbs they use are Anti-fungus, not poisonous to the body, only to the fungus.

For convenience sake, we grind the herbs, put them in capsules, and call them FNG Care™ and Blood Toner.

Maduromycosis

Another tumor forming fungus comes from India. It is called maduromycosis. Again, take the alfalfa seed herbal combination listed above and add emu oil so your trouble can be solved. Cut out sugar from your diet. Follow Dr. Otto Warburg's diet in the beginning of this book. Maduromycosis is known to make water filled tumors which surround a vital organ as the liver, intestines, even arteries. Please see a physician now, because it grows so fast.

Prostate Cancer

There is a special fungus which attacks the prostate. The organ swells and is in pain, the entire body feels sick, listless, hopeless and in despair.

Prostate cancer needs 2 herbal combinations along with milk compresses:

1. Candida Formula #2™, tansy, clay, milkweed, cramp bark, goldenseal leaves, blessed thistle

2. Mens Special®, saw palmetto berries, black walnut leaves, cornsilk

For the compress, dip a towel in warm milk. At bedtime, make a diaper of the milk soaked towel. Secure bed with plastic or a warm blanket. Follow these instructions for a week. Continue with herbs as indicated and cut down on fried foods.

Prostate trouble can affect men of any age. You do not need to be over 60 to be concerned about the prostate gland. In fact, a good time to start thinking about prostate health is long before those silver hairs emblazon your head. Young men in their early 20s have had bouts with prostate inflammation, much to their surprise.

The prostate gland is a firm, partly muscular, partly glandular body positioned beneath the bladder. Encircling the urethra, it squeezes out fluids which are ingredients in semen. This is where most male genitourinary problems occur. Three of the most common are prostatitis, benign hypertrophy and cancer.

Signs of Prostate Trouble

- **Urine retention**—The inability to empty the bladder because of a constricted urinary tract from enlarged prostate.
- **Incontinence**—Involuntary urination resulting from excessive urine in small amounts. There is also urge-incontinence or urgency which is the desire but inability to urinate.
- **Polyuria**—Frequent urination due to the bladder muscle becoming overdeveloped in trying to push urine through the impeded urethra producing an overactive bladder. This may indicate bladder failure is imminent.
- **Strangury**—Slow, painful urination accompanied by spasms of the urethra and bladder.
- **Nocturia**—Frequent urination during the night due to the bladder being full as the urinary passage is blocked with an enlarged prostate.

Prostate cancer is the third most common cancer in men just behind lung cancer and colon cancer. Almost

90 percent of prostate cancer goes undetected until it has gone beyond the most easily treated stage. Early signs of prostate cancer have the same symptoms as BPH—blood in the urine, difficulty in urination, strangury or nocturia. A cancerous prostate changes from a rubbery, firm consistency to a wood-like consistency upon examination. Venereal disease and recurring prostate infections have been linked to prostate cancer. Prostate cancer does not appear to be hereditary.

Diet plays an important role for this type of common cancer as well as other prostate disorders. *Men who have had a vasectomy are three times as likely to contract prostate cancer than men who have not had a vasectomy,* according to the August 1989 issue of the *Medical Tribune.* Surgery is a common treatment for prostate cancer and confirmation of prostate cancer should be done by a physician. Men over 45 should have a thorough prostate examination every 3 years.

There Are Options

Prostate problems can be serious. Luckily, there are many known natural remedies and preventions. Many of the herbs and foods that have been used for centuries are common in unrelated cultures. It is important to consult a health practitioner or physician for serious conditions such as cancer.

Herbs for Prostate

Saw Palmetto—This is a very common herb used for prostate health which may reduce inflammation, pain and throbbing. Although saw palmetto is native to North America, European research links it to reducing the size of the enlarged prostate. The oil found in the berry of the plant contains sterols, solid steroid alcohols, and various saturated and unsaturated fatty acids which are used medicinally in a purified fat soluble extract. One theory on hypertrophy is that excessive dihydrotestosterone (DHT), a derivative of testosterone, accumulates in the prostate. This causes the prostate cells to grow at an excessive rate, enlarging the gland. Saw palmetto prevents the conversion of testosterone into dihydrotestosterone, thus controlling the DHT levels and maintaining a healthy balance to the prostate. Tests have shown saw palmetto to reduce the frequency of nocturia, increase urine flow and reduce residual urine.

Cornsilk—The main action of cornsilk is its remarkable diuretic properties helping with urine flow when the urethra is constricted by an enlarged prostate. The active part of cornsilk is the gummy substance which contains fatty acids, menthol, glycosides, thymol, saponins, sugar, steroids, vitamins C and K and more.

Pumpkin Seed—This is one of the more fascinating herbs/foods for the prostate because it is cross-cultural. The native American Indians and native Africans have valued pumpkin seeds for the treatment of enlarged prostate. In Eastern Europe pumpkin seeds have been a common snack which gives some energy. There is also very little history of prostate problems from this part of the world. Other findings show pumpkin seeds to have cytotoxic characteristics helpful in fighting cancer induced prostate enlargement. The seed contains an antiparasitic compound also able to counteract cell division which may be responsible for treatment of BPH. Pumpkin seeds contain zinc which is an important nutrient for the prostate. (Raw pumpkin seeds are the most effective for any of these health properties.)

Black Walnut—Commonly known as a vermifuge or antiparasitic herb (which may work similarly to pumpkin seeds in the inhibition of cell division in the prostate), Hanna Kroeger has found black walnut to be helpful to the prostate, especially when used with diuretic herbs.

Parsley—Great Diuretic. Parsley contains apiol and myristicin and and stimulates urination and gives relief from urine retention.

Kelp—The people in Asia have used kelp for a long time in treating genitourinary tract disorders. Daily ingestion of kelp has been found to gradually reduce an enlarged prostate and alleviate painful urination, providing essential elements and relieving glandular congestion by supporting an exchange of body fluids.

Zinc—This mineral has been found to be beneficial in counteracting prostate enlargement and some studies show how zinc may inhibit the hormonal actions that cause prostate enlargement. The lack of zinc has been associated with prostatitis.

Vitamins

Vitamins are a good way of feeding the body what it needs to maintain good overall health and to overcome specific health conditions. One example of this is how the lack of vitamin A can cause distressful symptoms of the prostate gland as well as other significant repercussions in the body. Like vitamin E, vitamin A enhances the immune system and acts as an antioxidant. Vitamin B6 has been found to have anti-cancer properties which can be helpful to deter a cancerous condition in the prostate. Vitamin C in dosages of 1,000 to 5,000 mg per day promotes immune function and aids in healing. Vitamin E has been found to be very beneficial for the prostate. In fact, one doctor claimed he cured his prostatitis with 800 units of vitamin E daily, according to *The Big Family Guide To All The Vitamins* by Ruth Adams.

Do's and Don'ts

Other therapies can be combined with supplements and diet to get the prostate back to good health. Sitz baths (sitting in a tub of hot water for 15 to 30 minutes) once or twice a day increase circulation to the prostate region. Adding chamomile to the water can add a soothing effect. During healing, a chamomile enema once a week can cleanse the body of harmful acids. Include exercise such as walking into your daily routine.

Virus Tumors

Papilloma

One of the most widespread tumor formers is not a fungus but a very active virus called papilloma.

It is so widespread, so active, that in the main newspaper of Boulder, Colorado, a physician, Dr. Michele Manor, had the courage to report in two pages her research on papilloma.

It is the cause of cervical tumors, breast tumors, lymphoma, genital warts, and dysplasia.

Even endometriosis can be a papilloma virus. It can form brain tumors and anal tumors.

Dr. Manor reported that papilloma (called HPV) infects an estimated 10 to 20 million women between the ages of 19 and 49 in this country alone. It is one of the most common sexually transmitted agents, causing a pretty serious disease in infected women. Cervical tumors are the second most common tumors formed in women. Dr. Manor reports of 15,000 new cases each year in America alone.

The first step for checking yourself out is having an annual Pap smear. According to Judy Buck, women's health care nurse at the women's health care clinic at the University of Colorado's Wardenburg Student Health Center, "You can be infected with HPV and never have a symptom. It's very important all women have regular Pap smears because of this."

From a medical journal in Europe, I received my first hint that cervical cancer is caused by a virus.

In my search for an answer, I found the work of Dr. Sue Davidson, a gynecological oncologist with the Cancer Center at the University of Colorado Health Sciences Center in Denver. She said that the family of prevalent viruses collectively known as human papillomaviruses (HPV) are usually simple and painless viruses, however, they can become widespread and dangerous if not treated at once.

My granddaughter, after having her first healthy baby, showed an abnormal Pap smear. The advice of having her organs removed did not sound good to her. After three weeks on herbs and homeopathics, the Pap smear was totally normal and it is still normal 3 years later. Amazing!

Papilloma and Epstein-Barr

Two viruses coming together. These two are cyst-formers and tumor-makers. Treat like papilloma and add Epstein-Barr to it. It is a lot of pills, but the result is fabulous. It will take 2 to 3 weeks to clear the tumors. I still call it instant! Please add Dr. Johanna Budwig's cottage cheese formula. One pint every day for 2 weeks. Of course, you can also eat other good foods! Dr. Budwig is saying papilloma and other tumors can be helped with cottage cheese and oil, because this makes your own interferon.

Foundation Recipe Originated by Dr. Budwig

Put in blender or mix thoroughly by hand:

1 cup cottage cheese
2 tablespoons walnut or almond oil

This mixture is the foundation recipe and can be varied.

- Add finely grated horseradish. Serve with potatoes, buckwheat, and/or stewed carrots.
- Add tomatoes or tomato puree to taste. This is very delicious with rice, bulgur, or rye bread.

- Add chives, onion, parsley (finely cut) or paprika (finely cut).
- Make a colored surprise by adding to one part of cream cheese, tomato puree, or beets, a second part color with greens such as spinach, and a third part color with egg yolk. Arrange nicely and decorate with cucumber, tomatoes, radishes, etc.
- Heap the foundation recipe on lettuce leaves and top with a peach or apricot.
- As a dessert, use the cottage cheese sweetened with honey. Add a banana, a grated apple and some oat-flakes on top.
- Add honey, filberts, walnuts, almonds, all finely cut. Do not use peanuts. This is terrific for the center of a variety fruit plate. It is a whole meal!
- Make a little basket of the orange by scraping the inside out and adding honey to the foundation recipe. For parties, fill orange-basket with sweetened recipe.
- Use as salad dressing thinned with sour milk or thin cream. Add tarragon, parsley, paprika, rosemary or any herb or spice. Also add vegetable salt and a little lemon juice and more oil. It tastes delicious.
- The above salad dressing goes well with endive or white cabbage. Wild roses can be added to any salad. Cut them just before they are in full bloom.

These recipes are also terrific to eliminate scar tissue.

Herpes

Combined with other viruses, herpes can cause tumors. Herpes simplex viruses present a special problem in biology because they cannot be classified as living organisms yet they are able to invade living cells and direct the genetic machinery of these cells to reproduce the viruses. When the host cells become full of the virus, the cell bursts and dies. This is why the virus can cause deadly disease in spite of being so simple.

Viruses are much smaller than cells. Each type of virus is suited to its own type of host cells. For example, hepatitis prefers the cells of the liver. Herpes simplex prefers nerves and skin cells. Therefore, we have very few virus fighters. The anti-HIV drug, AZT, is a sophisticated tool of the 20th century. We are still without one for smallpox, chicken pox, measles. The herpes family consists of more than 40 distinct types of viruses that are found in every living animal. These viruses are classified together because they look the same. Here are a few viruses which appear:

Herpes Simplex: Cold sores, fever blisters on face, mouth, and lips. HSVI.

Herpes Simplex II: Usual cause of genital herpes, which is classified as a sexually transmitted disease.

Herpes III: Chicken pox, shingles. Also called varicella-zoster virus.

Herpes IV: Epstein-Barr virus. The major cause of infection. Mononucleosis, Chronic Fatigue Syndrome.

Herpes V: Cytomegalo virus, CHV. Virus causing hepatitis or mononucleosis.

VI, VII, VIII: All herpes viruses are connected with the immune system, especially AIDS and Kaposi's sarcoma.

Herpes virus is directly linked to a low functioning immune system. However, the strength and power of the herpes virus is many times aggravated because of our troubles with chemical vibration. As mentioned earlier, the herpes virus can cause tumors, as in Kaposi's sarcoma, associated with KSV, a tumor herpes. Also in tumors which occur in people with AIDS.

Ways to Help

We have to build our immune system. No sugar, caffeine, or food additives. We have to help ourselves with plenty of greens, grains, and low-fat protein. No smoking, and let's try to not overdo it on the alcohol.

If you let these things go untreated, the situation can escalate into cervical cancer. Women in their 30s or 40s are most in danger of this. If not caught early, one faces the very serious situation of hysterectomy, radioactive implants, and chemotherapy.

Unfortunately, we know very little about how the body works against this virus, though it is known to be the root cause of most cervical cancer and lymphoma.

Check for pancreatic flukes, liver flukes, blood flukes, and protozoa. The diet should be Dr. Budwig's diet as described earlier.

Retrovirus

The Newcomer

Retroviruses are RNA viruses. They are smaller than DNA viruses and they lump together in geometrical patterns. Retroviruses are originally found in animals such as mice and apes. They are a common virus to these creatures and one that does not hurt them. However, when found in humans, the results can be serious and devastating.

Retrovirus and Humans

Science was not aware of such a deadly virus until a tragedy starting in the 1950s. In an attempt to inoculate people for polio, a vaccine was cultured by using the kidneys of monkeys in which the retrovirus was present. This vaccine was administered directly into the bloodstream of 98 million Americans who unknowingly received the retrovirus called "Simian 40" or "Sim 40."

Retrovirus in humans can become active immediately or lay dormant for many years. It has been found dormant in regions of the nervous system for periods up to 30 years. It has been found hidden in areas of the lymphatic system and commonly appears in the blood. Little is known about what causes the retrovirus to act up but we do know that it has a disastrous effect on the immune system and can reveal itself as the common cause of many diseases. It appears that this condition is more widespread than recognized. In this age the retrovirus epidemic has claimed over one hundred and twenty-five million lives of men, women and children in Africa. This disaster is the result of a chicken pox disease vaccine that has inflicted many with what they term "Slim Disease." In Western countries, retroviruses, in combination with other viruses and fungi, cause several life-threatening afflictions.

> HEPATITIS C (Non A or B)
> ADULT T-CELL LEUKEMIA
> HAIRY CELL LEUKEMIA
> LYMPH CELL LEUKEMIA
> PERIPHERAL T-CELL LYMPHOMA
> NON-HODGKINS LYMPHOMA
> BREAST CANCER
> LUPUS
> MULTIPLE SCLEROSIS
> BRAIN TUMORS

There is a retrovirus kit consisting of herbs, homeopathics, and herbal capsules. It is useful for individuals whose T cell count is normal, but who have been infected with a retrovirus. This kind of virus is basically a strand of RNA, with an outer protein wall and outer lipid membrane.

Retroviruses replicate and mutate, and typically change into other forms, according to the environment they are in. This allows the virus to escape destruction. They are individual-specific; in other words, everyone has different forms of retroviruses.

Of all the viruses, retroviruses are the most feared because they can stay dormant for many years. They strike when the system becomes low in energy. They are unique in that they contain an enzyme call "reverse transcriptases." The HIV virus, for example, is said to mutate 13 to 15 percent per year. The retrovirus kit deactivates retroviruses.

Some studies have shown that in the presence of parasites, retroviruses take on the form of HIV.

Retroviruses are found in the following: lentivirus (ape virus), simian 40 (ape virus), HIV I and II, hepatitis C, adult T cell leukemia, and non-Hodgkin's lymphoma. When in combination with other viruses and fungi, retroviruses are found in: lymph cell sarcoma, T cell lymphoma sarcoma, peripheral T cell lymphoma, lupus, multiple sclerosis and hairy cell leukemia.

How Does This Virus Work

When a virus targets a cell to infect, it attaches itself to the outer membrane of the cell. From here the core of the virus, which contains all of the genetic information, penetrates and enters the cell. Once inside the cell, the virus uses the host cell and manufactures what it needs; a copy of its own genetic information and the proteins necessary for its survival.

Genetic Variability

A retrovirus has the unique ability to change its genetic make-up. This mutation causes a change in the virus particles called a genetic drift. These changes can occur both in the single individual and from person to person. These constant genetic changes allow the virus to escape immune destruction and make it difficult for an effective vaccine to be developed.

That means that the retrovirus can change according to the medium of the host. Therefore it is presented to us in many forms.

Retro-RNA Animal Virus

It appears that this condition is much more widespread than recognized.

It is found in:

Lentivirus (Ape virus)
Simian 40 (Ape virus)
Hepatitis C (Non A-Non B)
Adult T Cell Leukemia
Non-Hodgkins Lymphoma

In combination with other viruses and fungi, the retro-virus can also be found in:

Lymph Cell Sarcoma
T Cell Lymphoma Sarcoma
Peripheral T Cell Lymphoma
Lupus
Multiple Sclerosis
Hairy Cell Leukemia

Dr. Nieper, from Germany, stated that in breast cancer and also prostate ailments, retrovirus is frequently found.

It is also found in:

HIV
HIV II
HIV III
AIDS

Retrovirus turns into HIV and AIDS under the influence of hookworm, giardia, and amoeba. (Dr. Gallo and co-worker Anita Agarwal.)

Retroviruses change into multiple sclerosis and lupus if nickel and lead are in the body.

As we understand all these diseases have a common cause. Therefore, they can respond to the same basic formula.

To my mind came professor Dr. Brauchle's words. He said, "Miracles happen but you have to work hard for them." This miracle is the most important one ever. How I appreciate this.

Thank you Father in Heaven.

This formula is available now. Since all mentioned modern diseases have the same denominator—retrovirus—try this non-toxic gift from Heaven.

Reports

Alan Weaver said: After one week something changed in me. I saw nature differently. The sky was as blue as I remember when I was a boy. The leaves on the tree greener and the flowers so beautiful in color and design. A veil was lifted from my eyes.

Iris reported: After the sixth day, I could not keep my eyes open. I slept and slept. My tight muscles relaxed. No more shoulder pain, no more back pain.

A medical man bought several sets for his clients. He kept track of the results and to his amazement (and to mine) the retrovirus kit was building T cells in every one of his clients. This brave physician had to discontinue his research for fear of our present establishment.

To rebuild your body see a nutritionist.

New Formula for Tumors

From France comes a specific formula called Hydrazine Sulfate. It is said to have terrific results in the management of any type of tumor. We cannot buy it here and I can only write what friends in Europe report. After many weeks of prayer to our Lord to give us herbs for healing the afflicted, one morning when I woke up I found it written with my handwriting on my desk. I don't remember having been up and writing this one down.

Here it is:

HPX Formula™
Olive leaf
Echinacea root
Chaparral leaf

It takes the place of Hydrazine Sulfate, which kills viruses. Plus, it is stronger and non-toxic.

In Spite Of

There is a famous statue of Christ in Mexico which bears the strange name "In spite of." The artist Garcia lost his right hand in an accident. He had only finished the statue halfways when the accident happened. Wholeheartedly he determined himself to learn to carve with his left hand. And through his persistent effort the statue was finished. Better perhaps than he would have done with his right hand. For this reason the statue was called "In Spite Of." In spite of the fears and doubts building up in your life, if you are searching for God, if you are praying to God, truly and wholeheartedly, in spite of, you will be well.

CHAPTER IV

CHEMICAL AND METAL POISONS
In the Management of Tumors

These poisons create a medium in which parasites thrive. There is not one tumor-forming trouble that not only has poison, but also worms, flukes, protozoa, and other parasites. The worst parasites in tumor disease are roundworms. It eminates four different toxic chemicals which poison the body so much that there is no resistance left. These poisons, once in the bloodstream, have the same showing in the laboratory as a true tumor would show. It bluffs us.

Releasing Poisons

Hippocrates:
Diseases do not fall on us all of a sudden, diseases develop slowly by our daily sins against nature. After the accumulations of enough wrongdoings the body breaks down in disease.

Professor Dr. Katase, Osaha:
We have to fulfill a mission in regards to nutritional therapy. We have to secure the foundation of life of humanity now and for the coming season.

Professor Dr. Halden:
Comparatively few illnesses are of natural origin. Most illnesses are man-made.

Professor Dr. Kollath:
Lead is a protoplasmic poison, which means it interferes with the proper life-energy-enzyme exchange in the

living body. It is amazing how beautifully our system is able to take this lead poison. Everyone has it, only a few people in very isolated places in the mountains or prairies are free from lead intoxications.

There is to be considered (1) the amount of lead in our system, and (2) the tolerance factor of lead and other metals such as arsenic, cadmium, mercury and copper. This tolerance factor differs in everyone. Some people sponge in more arsenic than others, some sponge in more lead, or aluminum-lead or mercury. I found that red-headed people are prone to take in more copper than others and orientals more mercury. The fair people sponge in more lead or lead aluminum, and men more cadmium than children or women. Also, the individual tolerance level differs widely. Children and adults under emotional stress have an affinity to arsenic. (See the excellent studies from Japan on "Leukemia—Emotions and Arsenic Poison.")

Universal Remedies to Remove Metal Poisons

1. Mix 2 tbs. pumpkin seeds (ground) and 1 tbs. okra powder. Add ½ tsp. cayenne pepper. Take 1 tsp. of mixture with about 1 tbs. of rhubarb sauce, 3x daily for 10 days. *(Most effective with lead, arsenic, platinum, gold, and mercury.)*

2. Eat zucchini and green beans exclusively for three days.

3. Eat squash and strawberries. *(Most effective for arsenic poison, especially good for smokers.)*

4. Boil 3 lbs. of green beans in water until done. Add 2 lbs. finely chopped celery and 4 lbs. coarsely cut zucchini. Boil another 5 min. or until zucchini is done. Remove from fire and add 3 bunches of finely chopped

parsley. Season with spice. Eat only this for three days, make more if finished before three days. When reheating take only a portion from the refrigerator. Eat as often as you want. Drink parsley tea or willow leaf tea as a beverage. *(Most effective in removing metals lodged in glands and nerves.)*

5. An herbal remedy composed of pumpkin seed, okra, rhubarb root, capsicum, peppermint, and dulse also known as Metal X™.

6. Sulfur baths in natural springs or via granules, tablets or powders added to the bath water. *(Most effective for lead, arsenic, platinum, gold, and mercury.)*

7. Add 7 oz. liquid Clorox to warm bath in good sized bathtub. Bathe 10–15 min. *Note: not everyone can take Clorox baths, so check by soaking feet in a weak solution (1 tsp. to one gallon of water).*

8. Make a mixture of 4 oz. cranberry juice and 4 oz. distilled water. Take mixture 4x daily for 3 days, then wait 5 days and repeat.

Herbicide

Herbicide contains dioxin. Dioxin is Agent Orange. This broadleaf defoliant was used in Vietnam. It is used, so our lawns will not have dandelions or other broadleaved healing plants.

All poisons make a medium in which parasites, flukes and worms thrive. Dioxin however takes the cake. It binds these scavengers so tightly that ordinary anti-parasitic measures do not work. You have to have dioxin antidote with it.

Chart of Metal Poisons

Aluminum

Common Source

Aluminum cookware, canned food and soda, foil, etc., antiacids, aluminum sulfate baking powders, toothpaste, soft water, and antiperspirants.

Effect/Symptoms

Settles in brain (neural tissue).

Symptoms include: dryness of mouth, stomach pain, stomach ulcers, hard stool and/or with small hardened pieces ("fecal stones"), pain in spleen area, forgetfulness, children cry a lot, kidney problem—esp. the right kidney, and cell oxidation inhibition.

Extreme toxicity leads to: gastrointestinal irritation, colic, rickets, and convulsions.

Suggested Help

Protect with: Vitamin E, C, Metal X™.

Help with: Aluminae 6x-12x, or Co Enzyme International.

Arsenic

Common Source

Household and garden pesticides, insecticides via chemical called arsenoxide (both use and manufacture process). Coal burning, tobacco smoke, defoliants, metal smelting, manufacturing of glass, dental compounds for root canal fillings.

Effect/Symptoms

Settles in the muscles and the brain (dislodging phosphorus).

Symptoms include: sweet metallic taste, garlicky odor to breath and stool, constriction of throat, difficulties in swallowing, burning sensation (inflammation) in eyes, throat and chest, enlargement of tonsils, muscle spasms, pain in muscles of the back, adjustments to spine do not "hold."

Extreme toxicity leads to: mild gastrointestinal disturbances, anorexia, low grade fever with changes in white blood count, weakness (fatigue, listlessness, low vitality), brittle nails, loss of hair, skin color changes, dark spots, localized edema, and nervousness. *Since arsenic has a constricting effect on the muscle structure, and loves to lodge in muscles,* **the most outstanding symptom is the constant backache.**

Suggested Help

Protect with: Iodine, selenium, sulfur bath, amino acids, Vitamin C.

Help with: Arsenicum 6x, or Harpagophytum tea, or Tea with equal portions of quassia, white oak bark, and goldenrod. Drink 2 cups daily.

Chart of Metal Poisons

Cadmium

Common Source

Industrial exposure (e.g., from activities involving electroplating, low melting alloys, solders, batteries, pigments, barrier in atomic fission control, etc.), dental partial dentures, tobacco leaves, tobacco smoke, welding, paints, oxide dusts, contaminated drinking water, galvanized pipes, pigments, contaminated shellfish from industrial seashores.

Effect/Symptoms

Settles in heart and right kidney, and effects proper functioning of several enzymes.

Symptoms include: Pneumonitis, vomiting, diarrhea, loss of calcium in bones, deterioration of heart and blood vessel structures, and prostration.

Extreme toxicity leads to: Hypertension, kidney damage, loss of sense of smell (anosmia), emphysema, and decreased appetite.

Suggested Help

Protect with: Zinc, calcium, sulfur bath, amino acids, paprika, Vitamin C.

Help with: Cadmium-X 12x-30x

Copper

Common Source

Copper pipes and cooking utensils.

Effect/Symptoms

Settles in brain and ovaries.

Symptoms include: Burning sensation in throat and tonsils.

Extreme toxicity leads to: Wants to open hands all the time.

Suggested Help

Help with: Cuprum, or Zinc with B6

Gold

Effect/Symptoms

Tingling through system.

Suggested Help

Help with: Aurum

Chart of Metal Poisons

Graphite ─────────────────────────────

Common Source
Pencils, tires, lubricants.

Effect/Symptoms
Settles in heart.

Extreme toxicity leads to: Sense of numbness all over body.

Suggested Help
Help with: Graphite (homeopathic), or
   Breathe in steam of poppyseeds, and drink poppyseed tea.

Lead ──────────────────────────────────

Common Source
Paints, water pipes, tin cans, insecticides, motor vehicle
   exhaust (leaded gas), tobacco smoke, "moonshine" whiskey,
   newsprint & colored ads, hair dyes and rinses, dolomite, soft
   coal, leaded glass, pewter ware, pesticides, pencils, fertilizers,
   pottery, cosmetics, tobacco smoke, polluted air. Is a
   protoplasmic poison found in bleached white sugar.

Effect/Symptoms
Settles into liver, kidneys, spleen, and bone marrow.

Symptoms include: abdominal pain, anemia, enzyme poisoning,
   lowered osteoblast (bone) production, lowered blood
   formation, blockage of enzymes at cellular level, and lesions
   of the central and peripheral nervous system. *The central
   nervous system lesions result in behavioral problems such as
   hyperactivity in children.*

Extreme toxicity leads to: weakness, listlessness, fatigue, pallor,
   abdominal discomfort, constipation, hyperactive children,
   mad and weakened condition, lack of will power, lack of
   abstract thinking, lack of mental capacity, tooth decay,
   allergic reactions to food and environment, increases in
   diabetes and multiple sclerosis. **Lead is a protoplasmic
   poison, which means it interferes with the proper life-
   energy-enzyme exchange in the living body.**

Suggested Help
Protect with: Sulfur bath, amino acids, Vitamin C, E, calcium
   iron.

Help with: Plumbum, or
   Boil 3 teasp. whole cloves in 1 qt. cranberry juice for 20 min.
   Stir and add 3 qt. more juice. Now add 1 tsp. cream of tartar.
   Stir. Drink 5 oz. 3x daily. For children 3 oz. 3x daily for
   12–15 days. Then do it once a week.

Chart of Metal Poisons

Lead (continued) _____

Suggested Help

Tea using using mixture of: 6 oz. basil, 1 oz. rosemary, 1 oz. hyssop, 1 oz. boneset. Drink 1 cup 3x daily, or make

Tea using mixture of: Cloves and Vitamin C, or

Red Cabbage, or

Chamomile tea (to rebuild calcium after removing lead).

Mercury _____

Common Source

Manufacture and delivery of petroleum products, fungicides (for grains and cereals), fluorescent lamps, cosmetics, hair dyes, barometers, thermometers, amalgams in dentistry, salt water fish caught in contaminated waters, medications (diuretics).

Effect/Symptoms

Settles in liver, spleen, kidneys, intestinal wall, heart, skeletal muscles, lungs, and bones.

Symptoms include: Loss of appetite and weight, severe emotional disturbances, tremors, blood changes, inflammation of gums, chewing and swallowing difficulty, loss of sense of pain. Cell destruction, blocked transport of sugars (energy at cell level), increased permeability of potassium, convulsions, irregular heart beat, kidney, malfunction.

Extreme toxicity leads to: excessive salivation, metallic taste, blue line develops along the gingival margin, gums become hypertrophied, bleed easily and are sore, and teeth become loose. Tremors of the eyelids, lips, tongue, fingers and extremities. Coarse jerky movements and gross incoordination interfere with fine movements such as writing and eating. Visual deterioration, and dysphagia (difficulty in speaking). Atrophy of the cerebellar cortex, and to a lesser extent the cerebral cortex occurs. Microscopic changes occur in the granular layer of the cerebellum, ganglion cells, and posterior columns.

Suggested Help

Protect with: Pectin, sulfur bath, amino acids, Vitamin C, selenium.

Help with: Mercurium, or Green algae

Chart of Metal Poisons

Nickel

Common Source

Used to make hardened fats. Commonly found in all margarines, as well as oils and fats labeled **hydrogenated,** meaning hardened vegetable oil. *Be sure to check labels* of all prepared foods for use of **hydrogenated** or **partially hydrogenated** oils, including breads, chips, cookies, candies, etc.

Effect/Symptoms

Settles in sinus, joints, and spinal column.

Symptoms include: backache, headache, stuffed up sinuses, listlessness, swollen joints (knee, wrist, and ankle), and painful cracking neck.

Extreme toxicity leads to: paralysis, overflow of blood to brain, and epilepsy.

Suggested Help

Protect with: 1 tbs. of poppyseeds with honey by mouth 2x daily, poppyseed cake.

Help with: Nickel (homeopathic), or

Breathe in steam of poppyseeds, and drink poppyseed tea, or

Apply poppyseed compress to affected area of body.

Silver

Common Source

Photography, dental fillings.

Effect/Symptoms

Extreme toxicity leads to: Cold numbness through heart region, heavy weight on hands and feet.

Suggested Help

Help with: Argentum

Tin

Effect/Symptoms

Extreme toxicity leads to: Cold, icy feeling throughout body, numbness of feet.

Suggested Help

Help with: Stannum

CHAPTER V

REMOVING WORMS AND PARASITES
In the Management of Tumors

As I mentioned already, worms and parasites like a toxic medium, such as a toxic colon or toxic bodyfluid. Americans are the cleanest people. They shower or bathe every day. Daily a bunch of clothes goes into the washer, so it is *not* uncleanliness that makes worm eggs develop into destructive scavengers. It is the toxic medium caused by chemically affected food surroundings. The pH changes so much that even foreign scavengers such as bloodflukes and amoebas develop. All worms and parasites eat the best of the best of our body. All worms and parasites make the worst toxic waste, so they can multiply quickly and take over the host. Every tumor patient has some form of worms, flukes, or parasites—that is the name of the game.

WORMS AND PARASITES

	Where found	Actions	What to do
AMOEBA	underdeveloped countries	attacks intestines liver eyes	go to physician, also homeopathic antidote
BLOOD FLUKES	underdeveloped countries parasites	attacks blood makes bloodclots strokes	see physician, also homeopathic antidote
FISH FLUKES	undercooked fish	cause skin trouble intestinal trouble	avoid all raw fish, homeopathic remedies

	Where found	**Actions**	**What to do**
GIARDIA	unclean water	diarrhea intestinal trouble	see physician, also homeopathics
HOOKWORM	horses, dogs and their feces	drinks up to ½ cup blood every day, anemia	see physician, also homeopathic remedy
INTESTINAL FLUKES	origin unknown	makes lots of mucous, sinus trouble	see physician, also homeopathic remedy
LIVER FLUKES	water plants growing in polluted water	stimulates serious liver trouble	see physician, also homeopathic
LUNG FLUKES	origin unknown	shortness of breath, anemia	see physician, add homeopathic
PROTOZOA	wide spread in all countries	simulates arthritis leukemia Hodgkin's disease and many others	cuprum Ipecac Protozoa in homeopathic form
ROUND WORM	widespread in all countries	calcium deficiency children and adults	see physician, herbs for adults felix and cina for children
SALMONELLA	spoiled food also in chicken and some eggs	intestinal disorders, diarrhea, fever	apple cider vinegar
SPECIAL X	unknown	nervous system	Herb tea
TAPEWORM	the king of all worms	eats a lot and makes lots of toxins	see physician, also herbs

	Where found	**Actions**	**What to do**
THREADWORM	often found combined with Dioxin	anemia, itching all over	take homeopathic drops and see physician
TOXOPLASMOSIS	cat feces	attacks fetus low blood sugar	2 drops oil of sassafras 2 times daily to the soles of feet
TRICHINOSIS	pork and undercooked meat	attacks lungs, brain, heart, soft tissues	3 drops oil of wintergreen on 1 teaspoon molasses 2 times daily for 3 months
WHIPWORM	origin unknown	combines with dioxin, nervous system	dioxin antidote with whipworm antidote

Lately, it was discovered, even announced on television, that a hemolytic parasite (blood parasite) was found in all cancer patients. It was so tiny, the announcer said, that many hundreds could live in a drop of blood. Very interesting, dear Channel 4 announcer. It is too bad you did not give us more help on the question, "What can we do about it?"

Calmyrna figs have in their skins and kernels a substance which rips the skin of worms. It would be wise to eat some figs once in a while, just to make the environment in the intestine sweet and undesirable for the creature to live in.

See my book, *Parasites: The Enemy Within.*

CHAPTER VI

NATURAL PRODUCTS
In the Fight Against Tumors and Cysts

As interest in alternative medicine is increasing, researchers are now investigating many natural products for their ability to both protect against and treat cancer. I believe it would be helpful to look at some of the products they are currently investigating.

Aloe Vera   Has antitumor acitivity and may help reduce the spread of cancer to other tissues.

Astragalus   Will stimulate the immune system and has some antitumor activity.

Berberine   This alkaloid found in various herbs such as goldenseal and Oregon grape has been investigated for its ability to induce cell differentiation in cancer cells.

Bovine and Shark Cartilage   This has been used to stop cancer tumors from invading healthy tissues.

Bromelain   This is an enzyme derived from pineapple. It has been used to induce cell differentiation in human leukemia cells.

Burdock   This herb has been investigated for its ability to force cancer cells to differentiate.

Coenzyme Q-10   May help stimulate the immune system, and induce remission in cancer patients.

Flax Seed   Reduced risk for breast and colon cancer and also has some anticancer activity.

Frankincense   A specific for fungus tumors.

Garlic   May help reduce the spread of cancer (metastasis).

Ginseng   Inhibits damage done by chemotherapy.

Green Tea   Stimulates the immune system and inhibits tumor cell growth.

Horse Chestnut   This herb has been used to stop the growth of new blood vessels by cancer tumors.

Licorice   The compound glycyrrhizic acid found in this plant has been associated with antitumor effects.

Limonene   This chemical found in citrus fruits may have antitumor activity.

Tomatoes   As poultice for 3 nights in a row for deep-rooted tumor. In Europe it was used in brain tumors. (Prof. Brauchle)

Turnips   For deep rooted tumors. For deep-rooted resentments.

Vitamin A   This nutrient helps produce cell differentiation in cancer cells.

Vitamins C & E   Aids the immune system, reduced damage by chemotherapy.

Herbal Formulas

Dr. Rudolf Breuss of Austria instructs his cancer patients to take the following juices, especially for fungus tumors:

Red beet juice	5 ounces
Carrot juice	12 ounces
Celery root juice	7 ounces
White radish juice	½ ounce

Minerals

Professor Dr. W. Haupke:

Fifteen years ago, trace minerals were almost unknown. Nowadays, our knowledge is profound enough to realize that trace minerals are vital for the human body. We know that certain illnesses develop out of lack of trace minerals.

Hippocrates:

Illnesses do not come over us from somewhere and all of a sudden. They develop slowly from our "daily wrongs" against nature. When there are enough "wrongs" built up, they appear all at once and suddenly.

Dr. Kuhl, M.D.

Vitamin and mineral deficiencies can lead to tumor and cancer formation.

Chloride

Chloride is a component of hydrochloric acid. It maintains the acid/base balance. There is a link between chlorinated water and cancer of the gastrointestinal and urinary tract, so supplements not recommended in the treatment of cancer or candida! Refined salt like Morton's is full of chloride not balanced with other minerals like sea salt! Eat sea salt only!

Germanium

Dr. Levine said that germanium "activates or substitutes for oxygen." Dr. Asai discussed its chelating effects on heavy metals like cadmium. Germanium seems to have a cancer pain relieving effect.

The little district of Daun, West Germany, is rested peacefully and quietly in the setting of the old Vulcanic Mountains of the Eifel.

The lush green meadows, the wind swept trees, the little farms, and the quaint villages do not look different than they do in other parts of the country, and yet, the Daun District is entering the limelight of the world.

In 1944, several researchers became aware of the fact that in Daun, there was no cancer to speak of. A district without cancer. And those that had cancer when they came there were healed when they lived there for six months or longer.

At first, the scientists examined the soil and plants of this area. Finally, they found that the water of this area was different. It contained more magnesium chloride than other waters. They found 0.45659 mg. magnesium chloride per liter of water. Magnesium chloride is an activator of many, many enzymes. It is also needed in the breakdown of protein to amino acids, the building stones of the body. Magnesium chloride is also known to activate the Ester complexes. Much later, it was found that it was not the magnesium, but another element. It was *germanium* which was unique as a trace mineral in the waters of the Daun. This water is distributed as Dunaris Healing Water. Researchers went on the hot line to find out all they could about germanium.

Germanium is used in the electromagnetic industry to guide and focus energies. "Wild energies" become tamed with germanium. When I place my hand on a growth, I feel energies boiling, dashing, whirling, rushing, without guidance in an unbelievable turmoil. Of all the nations, Japan is far ahead with her research on germanium and cancer. North Korea has a district (like Daun) where hardly any cancer is found. This area has a very high content of germanium in the water and plants. Ginseng from Korea has the ability to accumulate more germanium than any other plant, and therefore, is greatly appreciated for its healthful benefits.

Sick Koreans go to the woods and search for a lichen which they eat. They also place lichens on tumors to reduce the size and pain. This lichen is loaded with germanium.

Here in America, we have good sources of germanium also. We have a spring which has the same mineral content as Dunaris Healing Water. We have clays (in Wyoming) and best of all we have corn. The Blue Corn (Squaw Corn) and the Indian Corn (Colored Kernels) are the richest of all the corn varieties for minerals and trace minerals, including germanium. A scientist from Rocky

Flats was in such bad shape that death seemed just a few steps away. I asked him which foods he really liked. After a long while, he said, "the morning mush made out of corn is the only thing I can eat." So, I told him to eat blue corn mush, mornings, noon and night or whenever he felt like it. Two weeks later, he had discarded all food supplements, but ate mush, corn grits and mush again. A few weeks later he was strong and now, after years, is working full blast.

Germanium in a natural state is in sprouted alfalfa and other sprouts. It is also available in tablet form.

Potassium

Potassium maintains osmotic pressure inside cells. It activates cellular respiration as it is a catalyst in the release of energy, protein and glycogen synthesis. LOSS OCCURS IN CATABOLISM? Magnesium deficiency depletes potassium. It also helps maintain acid/base balance. This is highly recommended in cancer treatment. *Mix capsules or crush pills in water to take because they can burn your stomach lining. It is better to take frequent smaller doses than one large dose.*

Sodium

Sodium maintains osmotic pressure outside cells. It inhibits cellular respiration and washes out potassium in the amounts found in the American diet. It is part of the digestive juices and thus counteracts excess acidity. Use sea salt for a healthier balance of minerals.

Selenium

Still not enough studies have been made on selenium, the "new trace mineral" with lots of potential. Up to now we know that selenium is needed to:

1. fight infection
2. detoxify many common pollutants

3. protect the heart, especially when combined with Vitamin E
4. make beautiful skin and give good vision

It also has something to do with cancer treatment. It is not understood how selenium accomplishes all that and more research has to follow. In all cases given, it uplifts the outlook on life. The sadness, despair and melancholy which is often seen in cancer victims is miraculously lifted. These people can take a hold of themselves again. Selenium promotes deeper sleep. Selenium gives a restful mind and peace within.

Selenium joins with glutathione to become cathione peroxidase and destroys dangerous peroxides free radicals. Do not use too much selenium, take it only from natural sources.

The main supplies are fish and liver. Dr. Gerson gave his patients lots of liver to eat. Nowadays liver is only safe when the animal has had no stilbesterol in the feed. I am more inclined to eat seafood. Mushrooms, good eggs, onion, and garlic are rich in selenium. Wheat and wheat products (if the wheat is organically grown) are also good sources of selenium.

Dr. Gertard Schrauzer, Prof. of Chemistry at the University of California at San Diego, said: "Selenium is one of the most efficient agents in stimulating the natural defense system against cancer."

Sulphur

Sulphur, magnesium, and germanium are the stars of the cancer diet. They play a major role in B vitamin coenzymes and in deactivating free radicals. Many hundreds of liver enzymes contain sulphur as it is integrated into the structure of your entire body. It is a component of mucus and is indispensable to immune function. Sulphurasis, cruciferous vegetables such as cabbage, broccoli, cauliflower, etc., are being heavily promoted by the American Cancer Society as an adjunct to conventional treatment and preventative measure.

Zinc

Chronic diseases are characterized by long-term mineral deficiencies, with zinc deficiencies being most commonly found.

Why is zinc necessary?

Fifty-nine or more enzymes require zinc for their functions or as part of their structure. Zinc is essential in the elimination of carbon dioxide in cellular respiration. It is involved in RNA and DNA synthesis and the incorporation of methionine into protein. It helps protect fats from oxidation and mobilizes vitamin A from the liver. It assists in hormone metabolism. Zinc is needed for all wound healing—whether from trauma or surgery. It is also important for the proper function of the pancreas (insulin production), thyroid, thymus and the immune system. Zinc also counteracts heavy-metal poisons (lead, cadmium and others) and helps prostate function and the reproductive organs. It helps too in managing multiple sclerosis, in overcoming skin problems and for the prevention of cataracts.

Why are we so in need of zinc when plants have it? Reason: plants grown with chemical fertilizer and other chemicals are not producing the link to zinc absorption by the cells of the body, and that link need is *picolinic acid*. Picolinic acid has nothing to do with pickles or cucumbers; it is an enzyme-hormone. Without this the human body cannot utilize zinc. And that is "the missing link," ZINC PICOLINATE.

Remember, the earmark of chronic diseases is mineral and trace mineral deficiencies caused by zinc malabsorption. ZINC PICOLINATE is a breakthrough in nutrition as nothing before. Let's overcome chronic diseases!

The National Cancer Institute reported zinc along with magnesium as two factors that inhibit carcinogenesis.

Liver and sunflower seeds are rich in zinc. Small frequent doses are recommended.

Vitamins

Dr. Kuhl, M.D.:
Vitamin and mineral deficiencies can lead to tumor and cancer formation.

Dr. Kollath, M.D.:
Cancer is the end result of years of poor nutrition and an unhealthy life style.

Vitamin A

Two cancer researchers from the National Cancer Institute's 1974 symposium report that they were able to prevent cancer in the windpipe of laboratory animals by giving them supervised amounts of vitamin A. Furthermore, scientists report that the vitamin can even help reverse cancer proliferation, if the patient is treated early enough in the illness.

> *NOTE: "This offers hope for a natural source for protection and/or reversal of cancer, an increasingly common fatal ailment,"* said Thomas Maugh, Ph.D.

More Discoveries Announced. As reported in *Science* magazine (December 1974), other researchers have found that vitamin A has a definite anti-cancer role. Thomas H. Maugh, Ph.D., suggests that cells may be protected after exposure to cancer by the action of vitamin A. It is believed, says Dr. Maugh, that the vitamin helps to "medicate a return to normalcy" after the damage has taken place, and this protects against more full-blown "transformation" of the cell to malignancy at a later date.

Dr. Maugh:
Vitamin A alerts the body's own built-in defenses to help reverse the cell damage caused by the carcinogen

and therefore prevent the cell's eventual surrender to cancer. Furthermore, vitamin A helps the body's defense system destroy cancerous cells.

Vitamin B_{15}

The whole vitamin B complex group is needed to sustain good health. Nature intended to create all B vitamins in the small intestine but our mode of living does not justify the assumption any longer that all of us have sufficient B vitamins. We don't have to go to pills, we can take rice polishings (women) or brewer's yeast (men). But for many it becomes easier to swallow a pill than to stir, mix, splash, and make faces.

There are two outstanding vitamins which are rarely discussed: B_{15} and B_{17}. B_{15}, also called pangamic acid, is a special one. It brings more oxygen to the tissue. It opens up the veins, arteries and capillaries so more oxygen supply can be furnished to the cells. Vitamin E also is an oxygen supplier and oxygen saver, but it does it only for the inner organs such as the liver, pancreas, heart and lungs. The two are a perfect couple. In Russia B_{15}, A, and E are routinely given to people over 50 and for all kinds of illnesses. Since in most illnesses we deal with a lack of oxygen supply, this knowledge becomes tremendously handy. *See findings of Dr. Otto Warburg.*

Vitamin B_{17}

B_{17} is not a newcomer. It has been used for a long time. Researchers found B_{17} in over one thousand plants. In bitter almonds and apricot kernels; it is present in the most concentrated form, but millet and all seeds show B_{17} in appreciable amounts.

The Chinese used bitter almond tea for tumors as far back as 3,500 years ago. It has been used in the Eastern World for centuries as an extract, a tea, and an infusion. In Turkey apricot kernels are combined with figs and eaten as a special treat for cancer-sick folks.

The Greeks and Romans used bitter almond water medicinally and called it Amygdalarum amarum. As early as 1845, Fedor Inosemzov, the Russian physician, combined bitter and sweet almonds for two kinds of "fungus-like tumors."

In the year 1830, the chemist, Robiquot and Boutron isolated B_{17} also called Amygdalin in its pure form. Only seven years later in 1837, the Scientists Liebig and Woehler discovered that Amygdalin is split by an enzyme complex into:

1 Molecule of Hydrogen Cyanide
1 Molecule of Benzaldehyde
2 Molecules of Sugar

Guide to B_{17} Foods

Kernels or seeds of fruits. The highest concentration of vitamin B_{17} is found in nature in the form of bitter almonds, apples, apricots, cherries, nectarines, peaches, pears, plums, and prunes.

Beans: broad (Vicia faba), burma, chick peas, lentils (sprouted), lima, mung (sprouted), Rangoon, scarlet runner.

Nuts: bitter almond, macadamia.

Berries: (almost all wild berries): blackberry, chokeberry, Christmas berry, cranberry, elderberry, raspberry, strawberry.

Seeds: chia, flax, sesame, clover.

Grains: oat groats, barley, brown rice, buckwheat groats, chia, flax, millet, rye, and wheat berries.

In the Himalayan Mountains of Pakistan lives an isolated tribe of people. They live in a beautiful valley called the Hunzaland. Travelers reported that the Hunzakuts are very healthy. Their women at the age of eighty look as we do at forty years of age. This sparked the interest of physicians such as Dr. Allen E. Banik, an optometrist, who was accompanied by some of his companions. They travelled the lengthy and dangerous roads on foot and horse, and found what was reported to be true. These peoples' diet consisted of lots of apricots, vegetables, millet and other grains. After Dr. Banik and Renee Taylor published their book on the Hunzaland we all started eating dried apricots.

The next explorers also found that they cracked the seeds of the apricots, so we started to eat the seeds to keep our figures and health at age 40. However, nothing spectacular happened. Then I read a book from a nature lover who reported the fabulous scenery, with the gushing waters coming down from the high mountains which were white with minerals rushing through the entire territory of the Hunzaland. It was reported that the inhabitants treat this water like a holy spring. No garbage is thrown into it. They use the water only for their gardens and for their water supply in the houses. This pure water is loaded with calcium carbonate. Here lies the secret of the Hunzakuts' fabulous health.

Apricots provide enzymes.
Apricot kernels have B_{17}, the longevity factor of the cells. Calcium Carbonate, or lime water, is needed to make the enzymes in the apricot active so that this enzyme can assimilate vitamin B_{17}.

Whether B_{17} cures cancer or not is not for me to say, but it surely takes pain away. B_{17} brightens the dark days of a cancer victim. Patients are feeling better and happier. All cases are eating better and gaining weight and strength.

Dr. Dean Burk, head of the Cytochemistry Section of the National Cancer Institute, Bethesda, Maryland, said "B_{17} is non-toxic." After testing B_{17} on rats he said, "Aspirin tablets proved to be twenty times more toxic to the animals than Amygdalin."

Here is your homemade B$_{17}$:

  4 apricot kernels
  2 pieces dried apricots
  5 Calcarea carb., 6x homeopathic, or limewater

Chew this. Take the formula twice a day. It tastes wonderful. Everybody should have this treat, at least once a day!

Commercially, B$_{17}$ is called laetrile. There are two kinds of laetrile: one is female in nature and one is male in nature. Therefore sometimes it helps and sometimes it doesn't. The controversy is on. The natural product as indicated has both male and female aspects and the body picks what is needed.

Nutrition

According to the world famous cancer research physician, Dr. Hans Nieper of Germany: "In Germany it is a law. When someone has cancer, doctors must tell the patient that there are four alternatives:

  surgery
  radiation
  chemotherapy or
  nutrition

The doctor must explain nutrition to the patient, and the patient may take the choice."

What is "Correct Nutrition"

Many books have been written on this subject. In essence they contain the following:

  1. quality of food
  2. quantity of food
  3. proper preparation of food
  4. electromagnetic energy in food
  5. food combining

Quality of Food

The industrial treatments of natural foods has in no way increased the *quality of food*. The accumulative effects of chemicals, additives, and colorings are discussed at length in many pamphlets and books. The advantage of long shelf-life of cereals, flours, ready-made products, oils, fats, breads and other necessities of life carry a stigma of dark angels with them. The dark angels bring suffering and ruination of good health.

The terrible human suffering of added hormones to the feed of animals is rarely discussed. Chicken, eggs, milk and meat still carry the hormonal additives that can make large changes in the male-female relationship of humans. The delicate hormone balance is constantly upset. The very cell is in an uproar. Here are some experts speaking:

Dr. Kotshan (MD):

"Our civilization thinks and teaches that by beautifying natural foods, its quality could be improved. However, applying our advanced technology to food preparation, preservation, packaging and manhandling, the biological substance of our entire population is at stake."

Dr. Kollath (MD):

"The nutritional crisis in which we are now is something new in history. The change in the quality of food by taking natural substances away and replacing them with artificial additives will always denature the food value and serious consequences have to be expected."

Dr. Vollati also said:

"Denatured nutrition can destroy the best nation and, therefore, it should be in the interest of the government to protect its subjects from using denatured food."

The Preparation of Food

The *preparation of food* starts with shopping. Farmers Markets are the best. Here one can find a great selection of homegrown vegetables, delicious unsprayed apples, tree-ripened fruit, and berries of all kinds. The pure honey and fertile eggs!!! The chickens run and have exercise. They are fed grains and greens so you can taste the goodness of nature in every egg. But most of us have to go to Super Markets. The fruit was picked green for transportation's sake, particularly the tomatoes, which are usually tasteless. The colored oranges and the waxed cucumbers look beautiful. There again, we find industrialization for beauty's sake.

We know the dangers of pesticides, coloring, additives, and preservatives. We know that all these things have an accumulative, detrimental effect on the body's reserves. Alkaline Acid imbalance becomes a contributing factor to severe illnesses when enough poisons enter the tissues.

There are several proven methods to counteract the foreign substances in food, vegetables, milk, water, fruit and everything else consumed.

For many years the "Soma Board" has been on the market. This has kept many, many families in excellent health. It is made with herbs, crystals, magnetic alloids, and other items. It lasts for 16 years. Just place foods, milk and juices on or around it.

Detoxifying is a process of neutralizing chemicals and additives in food or liquids so they become harmless to the body. Detoxifying foods will not improve the mineral or vitamin content of such treated foods. Mineral deficient merchandise will stay that way; however, the small amount of minerals present can be assimilated completely.

The Body is an Electrochemical Energy System

This energy system needs fuel to function properly. It needs fuel that has energy to give. Foods that have been manhandled—canned and filled with additives, irradiated, microwaved and wrongly combined—will not release sufficient energies to keep us going. Nor will it keep our brain at high gear or keep us free from disease. "Disruption of cellular energy is what we label disease." I heard this sentence stated by a medical doctor and it hit me— this is heavenly truth!

Scientists tell us that the amount of food and fluid we take in is eliminated at the same ratio as ingested, ounce by ounce and pint by pint. What we live on is the electrochemical energy created—emanated from our food and fluids. If we continue to take in food which is low in electro-chemical power we lower our resistance. This means that we cannot ward off environmental poisons which are in water, air and food.

Today, we have to create a different way of eating and adapt a different lifestyle. Understanding kitchen chemistry is a must in order to keep our family alive and healthy. Dr. Parcels said: "The relation of foods one to another will greatly establish the electrochemical energies." She also said, "these energies need a slightly acid environment to function." If the environment is too *alkaline*, the *functions* of electrochemical energies will slow down or stop entirely depending on the amount of alkalinity.

Electrochemical energies are destroyed in over-cooked foods, old food, over ripe food, irradiated food and food that passed through a scanning machine in stores. The most important cause, however, is our habit of wrong food combination.

How to Combine Foods for Best Electrochemical Energy

Bread and cheese is a no-no.
Bread and meat is a no-no.
Bread and chicken is a no-no.
Macaroni and cheese is a no-no.

Citrus fruit and grains make a tough mucus in the stomach and in the sinuses; other fruits and grains will not do that. Sweet fruit is a desirable food but must be eaten as a meal or between meals. Only the apple is neutral and can be eaten with vegetables or meats. Apple sauce and stewed apples are fine.

DO NOT EAT FRUIT AND VEGETABLES TOGETHER. MEAT AND MILK IS A NO-NO.

Meats need vinegar used as a salad dressing (acids) to be prepared for digestion. If you drink milk with meats, the hydrochloric acid (HCL) is neutralized and the meat rots in the stomach.

Grains and meats are a very poor combination, so are grains and cheeses. Think of your sandwich at noon! You become tired and listless after a double decker!

Fruits are fine mixed, cut in cubes or whole, but do not eat nuts with it. If you put nuts with your fruit salad, your fruit salad has no vibration.

Carrots and peas mixed look so pretty and so inviting but it will not feed your body through the electrochemical function. It becomes a ballast.

THE APPLE IS THE EXCEPTION!
RICE IS AN EXCEPTION!

Apples in all forms can be mixed with vegetables. Rice can be taken with protein.

The electrochemical diet makes your life light burn brightly. Where there is light, the darkness has to disappear. The atomic influences, the chemicalization, and the metallic poison cannot easily disturb the balance in you. It is the way of survival.

A good dinner consisting of salad, vegetables, meat or chicken, and/or cheese, should never have a dinner roll with it. A dinner roll by itself may serve as a snack between meals or before bedtime. If you are in need of putting on weight, have a roll before bedtime with plenty of butter!

Dr. Kuhl's Cancer Diet

This researcher is very well known and his findings are well founded. The result is excellent. He improves cell respiration by taking cold pressed oils in salads, cottage cheese and in vegetables. He gives yoghurt, sauerkraut, cottage cheese, kefir, buttermilk, fermented vegetable juices, and in particular fermented beet juice. Vegetables and fruits should be organically grown, i.e., without spray or artificial fertilizers. Carbohydrates and sugar are not on the menu. Some eggs and fowl are permitted.

When you first get out of bed in the morning:
>   Drink diluted cherry juice
>   or lemon juice and water
>   or cranberry with lemon peel, soaked overnight.

Breakfast:
>   fruit and flax seed ground up
>   or, barley with honey, cream and fruit
>   or, millet cereal with cream and cottage cheese with oil
>   or, a slice of whole wheat bread

Juice for in-between meals. Beet or carrot juice.

Lunch:
>   Have cooked vegetables, a raw vegetable salad, and
>   fish, or chicken, or lamb.

Afternoon:
>   Fruit and whole wheat toast if desired.

Supper:
>   Have raw salad, rice, asparagus, yoghurt, vegetables. No
>   animal protein at night.

The reason for not having protein at night is: If you eat protein such as chicken, eggs, fish or meats, it takes the body 8 hours to break the protein down to amino acids. The building stones of the tissue are amino acids. The carrier of these valuable amino acids is the lymph system. At night the lymph system closes down to low function and the liver will dump the building stones into the cancer growth. When you eat protein at night you feed your cancer but starve your body.

Special Formulas

High Mineral Broth

Wash well and peel 2 quarts potatoes. Discard potatoes and use peel only.

To each cup potato peels add 2 cups of water.

Simmer 1 hour or until very soft. Mash well, drain off liquid.

Drink 4 oz. of liquid morning, and 4 oz. at noon.

Blood and Tissue Cleansing Plan

Start this diet plan with this thorough cleansing plan.

Repeat cleansing plan one day every other month.

Morning: 1 quart unsweetened grape juice

Noon: 1 quart orange juice (canned or fresh)
        2 thick slices *raw* onion

3 P.M.: 1 quart pineapple or prune juice

Evening: 1 quart grapefruit or orange juice (canned or fresh)
        2 thick slices *raw* onion

Blood Feeding

Clean well large turnips (rutabagas or yellow turnips when in season).

Dice into 1 inch pieces. Cover with distilled water. Simmer until soft.

Mash liquid in well and strain through very fine screen or cheese cloth.

Drink 1 quart of this liquid every day.

Under sterilized sanitation, this has been scientifically proven. The above formula if given intravenously—works like a miracle—used instead of blood transfusion—it never fails.

Calcium Normalizing Broth

1 teacup unprocessed bran. (consult your health food store.) Add

1 quart distilled water.

Bring to a boil over low flame, remove at once and let stand for 2 hours. Strain as you use. Sweeten with honey. Drink 8 oz. twice daily.

Digestive System Normalizer
Chop, grate or slice thin, 1 quart white or red cabbage. Add 1 quart water. Boil ½ hour or until soft. Draw off liquid. Use 4 oz. of liquid each day. Supplies vitamin U, Alkalime, sulphur, calcium, zinc, phosphorus, iron, copper, vitamins C, A, B_1, G.

Here are some hints on how to protect yourself against poisons.

—Drink catnip tea for arsenic poisoning.
—Drink mandrake root tea after you've taken poisoned water.
—Drink pokeberry tea for sodium fluoride poison.
—Put green grass in a bottle. Let it stand for two hours—This also binds sodium fluoride to the green.
—For fallout take a soda and salt bath.

The following recipe removes lead from your tissue:

1 gallon cranberry juice
2 tbsp. whole cloves
2 tsp. ground cinnamon
1 tsp. cream of tartar

DIRECTIONS: Boil the cloves in 1 quart cranberry juice for 20 minutes. Strain and add two tsp. ground cinnamon. Stir and add it to the rest of the cranberry juice. Now add 1 tsp. cream of tartar. Stir. Drink 5 ounces 3 times daily. For children, 3 ounces 3 times daily for 12–15 days. Then do it once a week.

CHAPTER VII

CYSTS

Breast Lumps

Breast lumps can be removed at an early stage, without surgery, by stimulating the lymph flow. Have the woman stand and have a second person, preferably the male energy of her husband, do the following: (for purposes of this example we will assume the lump is on the right side).

1. Stand on the right side of the standing patient. Put the spread fingers of the right hand on the right side of the sternum where the breast tissue attaches. Simultaneously put the spread fingers of the left hand on the right side of the spinal column, approximately parallel with the right hand. Hold for 60 seconds. Prayers for healing are entirely in order through these stages by both the subject and the practitioner.
2. While holding the left hand in the same place, move the right hand to a position directly in the armpit, with the spread fingers extending straight down out of the armpit. Again hold for 60 seconds.
3. Return to position one and hold for 60 seconds.
4. While holding the right hand in the same place on the right side of the sternum, shift the left hand to the position in the armpit and down from it. Hold for 60 seconds.
5. Return to position one and hold for 60 seconds.
6. Repeat this process 3 times a day until three days after the lump disappears. If the lump is on the left side, exchange the words right and left in the above instructions. If it does not disappear in three weeks,

the case is more advanced and needs different care, including the possible use of magnets or fungus removing herbs. Of course, there is always the possibility the lump is something other than a blockage of the lymph glands.

Left Hand   **Right Hand**

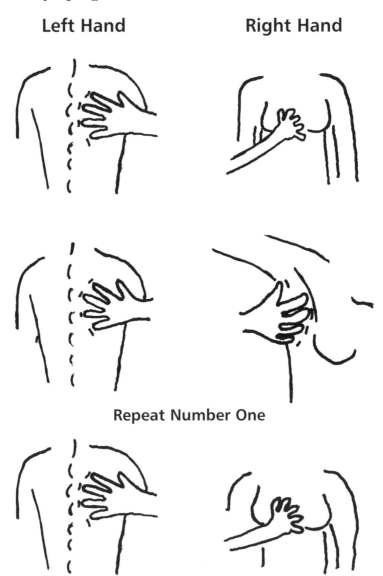

Repeat Number One

Left Hand   Right Hand

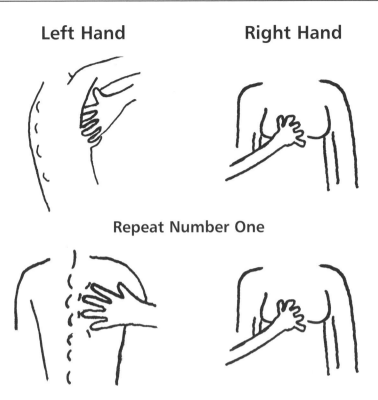

Repeat Number One

Every position should be touched for 60 seconds.

Cysts in Ovaries

Key position for the ovaries. Heal your ovaries by holding the points indicated in diagram. Very valuable in cases of tubular pregnancy. In that case, someone else should hold these points for 15 minutes.

Apply *Black Cohosh Tincture.*

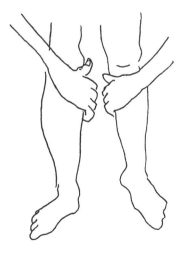

Herbal Formula for Cysts

CYT Formula™
Cottonwood Leaves
Grape Leaves
Chaparral

2 caps., 3 times daily

CHAPTER VIII

LEUKEMIA

Leukemia does not make tumors, so it does not belong to the tumor making diseases. It causes swelling of the lymph glands and spleen.

Leukemia and Its Management

I had the good fortune to be working as a registered nurse in Dresden, Germany, at a 2,000 bed hospital for natural healing which was headed by Dr. Brauchle. There he stated the following truth on leukemia: "Leukemia is not cancer of the blood." He taught that there are 3 causes of leukemia:

No. 1   The disintegration of the blood is caused by a malfunctioning of the Portal Vein System. The Portal Vein System is the system that draws the nourishment out of the food we eat and also converts Prana into life energy.

No. 2   Most leukemic cases are found in homes where husband and wife fight. Or in cases of divorce, or when the spiritual need of a child or an adult is not understood.
In short, it is a love situation. The Portal Vein System is extremely sensitive to emotions and will close shut if something is wrong emotionally.
Please have a happy table surrounding when you eat. No fighting, no shout outs, no ugly words. The poisons so created is a cause for the digestion to close down the Portal Vein's functioning.

No. 3   Most leukemic patients have a tailbone dis-
placement. Go to a chiropractor and have the tailbone put back in order. The tailbone is the pump for
the spinal fluid. If the pump is stuck, the spinal fluid
and also the cerebral fluid will not function. The tailbone also is taking care of the waste product of the
nervous system. (See below for instructions on *How
to Set the Tailbone.*)

IMPORTANT

Repeated nosebleeds in children should always be
treated by a physician. One to two years before a "blood
break down," a period of nosebleeds is experienced.

This is what we did in Professor Brauchle's hospital of
Natural Healing:

First the tailbone had to be set.

"The Happy Floor"

Nurses had to prepare and give the following delicious
drink to all leukemia cases. Besides the main kitchen in
the huge establishment, there was a diet kitchen on each
floor. We loved those diet kitchens. They were large,
handsome, and light, while the pharmacy department
next door was small, compact, and had only a small win-
dow. In the kitchen we prepared:

   1 pint white grapefruit juice
   1 pint freshly squeezed orange juice
   1 pint grape juice
   1 pint water with the juice of three limes
   1 pint water with the juice of two lemons
   1 pint frozen pineapple juice diluted
   1 pint papaya juice, diluted

Take 12 whole eggs and 6 egg yolks. Beat eggs very
thoroughly and mix into fruit juice mixture. Sweeten with
honey if needed. For a change of taste, you may add

frozen raspberries or strawberries. This was enough for two or three children a day, but an adult could drink that much without hesitation.

Adults should drink:
Beet juice—3 parts
Carrot juice—2 parts
Celery root juice—12 part

If celery root juice cannot be obtained, the first 2 juices alone are very, very helpful. 5 ounces 2x daily.

The following herbal tea in equal parts will help to open the Portal Veins.

melilot
calendula
St. John's wort

Leukemia is a serious disease, but there is *NO* fungus involvement.

Prof. Brauchle never lost a single case of a leukemia stricken child. Couldn't we try also? It takes only days to help.

How to Set the Tailbone

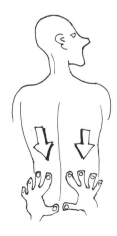

1

Put person on stomach and loosen the spine by light massage down- ward on both sides of the spine. Do it 3 times on each side.

Turn their head so it is facing you. Hold one hand over sacrum.

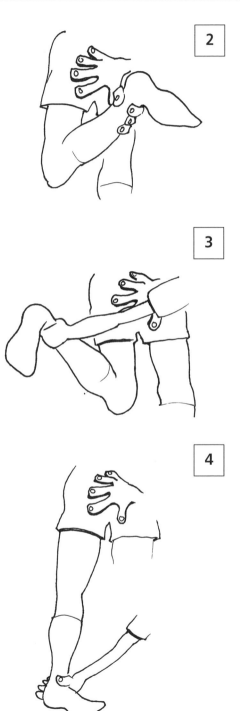

Lift the leg farthest from you, bend knee and bring it toward you (inside) and back to the middle. Do this 3 times. Now 3 times outside and back to the middle. Then down and back to the middle 3 times. Then up and back to middle 3 times.

Now turn their head the other way. Repeat: 3 times inside, 3 times outside, 3 times down and 3 times up.

Now lift leg by slid-
ing under thigh and
swing leg toward
you 1, 2, 3 times.

Now go to other
side of the person
and repeat all steps.

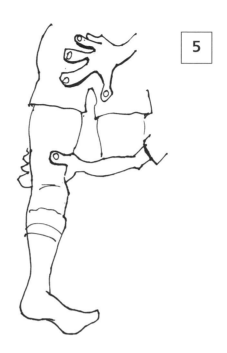

5

CHAPTER IX

THE SPIRITUAL FACTOR
In the Management of Tumors

This book would not be complete without this chapter, the spiritual part in the management of tumors.

Cancer stricken people go through the following emotional upheavals:

disbelief
anger
despair
giving up

When you are diagnosed as having cancer, you will have a great disbelief.

"I have no pain."
"I am a little more tired."
"I am overworked."
"But I do not have cancer."

Always seek a second opinion. Suppress your thoughts and feelings of doom by saying to yourself, "all things *are* possible to him that believeth." (Mark 9:23).

After the verdict of the second physician, I suggest that you change your diet as outlined and also straighten out your thinking. From a possessive thinking switch over to a freedom of unpossessiveness.

You do not possess your children. They are God's children and you are allowed to help them and feed them for awhile but they are God's creation. So is your husband. There is an abundance of God's love and God's work. So are you, a joy to God. John 20:27 says, "Be not faithless, but believing." Say constantly, "Yes Lord, I believe in the first stage of the discovery of cancer." Say these words constantly. As you believe in something, you also do something about it. And the change has to come in the wholeness of your being and the wholeness of your action.

When you arrive at the second stage, the stage of Anger, you will ask, Why Me? Why not my enemy. I have so much to do. Why has God given me this cross to bear. I honestly say good for you! Be angry, be mad, stamp your foot on the floor, kick your pillow, yell, run. Take the professional widespread concept, "you have cancer, you have to die," and rip it apart. Get ready to fight and fight well. Use the healthy power of your will! Will is an energy. Willpower is located in your forehead and next to it is the power of understanding. If you use willpower, you might come upon trouble; but with willpower comes understanding. The power of understanding goes into the depth of your being. Understanding goes to the intuitive power, which is God-centered. Will power and the power of understanding is expressed in the words, "not mine but Thy will be done." This is not a negative statement. Thy will O Lord is health, well-being, and happy accomplishments, so I will understand this and get well quickly to do His will on earth.

The third stage of your way downhill is despair. When you are in despair, your muscles contract and circulation is cut off. You start having pain. You think that this is the end of your life. Relax, relax. Ask for the power of strength and ask for the Divine Order of Christ. Your power of order is at your solar plexus. This solar plexus also is the vessel, The Golden Grail, through which new ideas, new inventions, new strength is arising. When this vessel is full of old junk, such as resentment, unforgiveness, disharmony, and negative emotions, the power of order cannot manifest. Clean out that stuff and start anew. As soon as you have cleared this vessel, Hope will enter. Where there is hope, life will enter. Where there is life, God holds your precious life in his hands and will give you strength, endurance, and love.

The last of the four stages is that one in which cancer patients will "give in." They sit there and wait for the hour to part from us. Oh dear beloved brother, dearest sister, only God knows the hour. We had a physician in class. He said, "I have seen miracles. I thought 'this breath is the last breath my fellowman is taking,' but it was not the last, but the first of a long life to come. Never give up."

My book *The Seven Spiritual Causes of Ill Health* will help you tremendously. On request, The Chapel of Miracles will send you healing prayers. Send handwriting and full name to:

Chapel of Miracles
7075 Valmont Road
Boulder, Colorado 80301

We all have intuitive power. We all have the sixth sense in order to find our paths in life. Please put this divine gift to work. If you are in doubt, have someone help you with muscle testing or dowsing.

This is what you do:

Ask a friend to muscle-test you on the following items.

Fungus:	Hard Tumor
Fungus:	Maduromycosis
Fungus:	Prostate
Virus:	Papilloma
Virus:	Papilloma & Epstein-Barr
Retrovirus:	A Virus and Monkey Poison

PEARLS FROM THE BIBLE FOR HEALING

PSALMS 3:3-4

But thou, O Lord, *art* a shield for me; my glory, and the lifter up of mine head.
I cried unto the Lord with my voice, and he heard me out of his holy hill. Sē'lah.

PROVERBS 17:22

A merry heart doeth good *like* a medicine: but a broken spirit drieth the bones.

ISAIAH 38:21

For Isaiah had said,
Let them take a lump of figs, and lay *it* for a plaister upon the boil, and he shall recover.

PROVERBS 24:13

My son, eat thou the honey, because *it is* good: and the honeycomb, *which is* sweet to thy taste.

When bleeding is present, read:

EZEKIEL 16:6, three times. The bleeding will stop.

Three times in a row, three times a day, say:
"By his stripes, thou shall be healed."

You will be amazed what a relief this is to you when you have pain.

Books by Hanna

 "Wholistic health represents an attitude toward well being which recognizes that we are not just a collection of mechanical parts, but an integrated system which is physical, mental, social and spiritual."

Ageless Remedies from Mother's Kitchen

You will laugh and be amazed at all that you can do in your own pharmacy, the kitchen. These time tested treasures are in an easy to read, cross referenced guide. (92 pages) ISBN: 1-883713-04-8

Alzheimer's Science and God

This little booklet provides a closer look by presenting Hanna's unique and religious perspectives. (15 pages) ISBN: 1-883713-10-2

Arteriosclerosis and Herbal Chelation

A booklet containing information on Arteriosclerosis causes and symptoms. (14 pages) ISBN: 1-883713-03-X

Free Your Body of Tumors and Cysts

Hanna brings together many natural techniques, including diet, herbs, vitamins, hands-on healing and more in a practical, understandable approach to growths and their relationships to parasites, cancer and leukemia. (77 pages) ISBN: 1-883713-18-8

Good Health Through Special Diets

This book shows detailed outlines of different diets for different needs. Dr. Reidlin, M.D. said, "The road to health goes through the kitchen not through the drug store," and that's what this book is all about. (90 pages) ISBN: 1-883713-14-5

Help One Another

It's the most complete compilation of Hanna's works to date; combining all the information from her 20 books with contributions from practitioners who worked closely with her. There are approximately 300 pages of Hanna's teachings on remedies, recipes, cleanses, foods, supplements and hands-on procedures. There is also an extensive index. A great resource! ISBN: 1-883713-19-6

How to Counteract Environmental Poisons

A wonderful collection of notes and information gleaned from many years of Hanna's teachings. This concise and valuable book discusses many toxic materials in our environment and shows you how to protect yourself from them. It also presents Hanna's insights on how to protect yourself, your family and your community from spiritual dangers. (53 pages) ISBN: 1-883713-15-3

Instant Herbal Locator

This is the herbal book for the do-it-yourself person. This book is an easy cross-referenced guide listing complaints and the herbs that do the job. Very helpful to have on hand. (109 pages) ISBN: 1-883713-16-1

Instant Vitamin-Mineral Locator

A handy, comprehensive guide to the nutritive values of vitamins and minerals. Used to determine bodily deficiencies of these essential elements and combinations thereof, and what to do about these deficiencies. According to your symptoms, locate your vitamin and mineral needs. A very helpful guide. (55 pages) ISBN: 1-883713-01-3

New Book on Healing

A useful reference book full of herbal, vitamin, food, homeopathic and massage suggestions for many common health difficulties. This book is up-to-date with Hanna's work on current health issues. (155 pages) ISBN: 1-883713-17-X

New Dimensions in Healing Yourself

The consummate collection of Hanna's teachings. An unequated volume that complements all of her other books as well as her years of teaching. (150 pages) ISBN: 1-883713-09-9

Old-Time Remedies for Modern Ailments

A collection of natural remedies from Eastern and Western cultures. There are more than 20 fast cleansing methods and many ways to rebuild your health. A health classic. (105 pages) ISBN: 1-883713-05-6

Parasites: The Enemy Within

A compilation of years of Hanna's studies with parasites. A rare treasure and one of the efforts to expose the truths that face us every day. (62 pages) ISBN: 1-883713-07-2

The Pendulum Book

A guidebook for learning to use a pendulum. Explains various aspects of energies, vibrations and forces. Now with an additional workbook section so you can apply this universal knowledge right away. (35 pages) ISBN: 1-883713-08-0